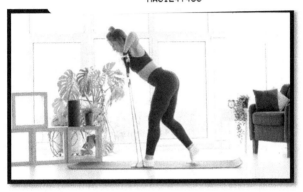

SINGLE BAND WORKOUT

By:

Kevin B DiBacco

DISCLAIMER

No part of this publication may be reproduced in any form or by any means, including printing, scanning, photocopying, or otherwise, without the prior written permission of the copyright holder. The author has tried to present information that is as correct and concrete as possible. The author is not a medical doctor and does not write in any medical capacity.

All medical decisions should be made under the guidance and care of your primary physician. The author will not be held liable for any injury or loss that the reader incurs through the application of the information contained in this book. The author emphasizes that the medical field is fast evolving with newer studies being done continuously, therefore the information in this book is only a researched collaboration of accurate information at the time of writing. With the ever-changing nature of the subjects included, the author hopes that the reader will be able to appreciate the content that has been covered in this book. While all attempts have been made to verify each piece of information provided in this publication, the author assumes no responsibility for any error, omission, or contrary interpretation of the subject present in this book.

Please note that any help or advice given hereof is not a substitution for licensed medical advice. The reader accepts responsibility in the use of any information and takes advice given in this book at their own risk. If the reader is under medication supervision or has had complications with health-related risks, consult your primary care physician as soon as possible before taking any advice given in this book.

"The information and advice contained in this book are based upon the research and the personal and professional experiences of the author. They are not intended as a substitute for consulting a healthcare professional. "

"The publisher and author are not responsible for any adverse effects or consequences resulting from the use of the suggestions, preparations, or procedures discussed in this book. All matters pertaining to your physical health should be supervised by a healthcare professional."

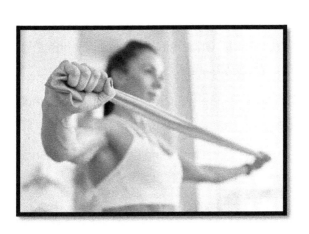

Table of Contents

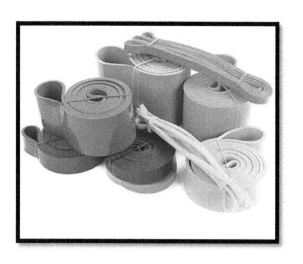

Kevin's Remarkable Journey of Strength and Resilience

Kevin's lifelong passion for powerlifting and fitness has been nothing short of remarkable. Though the journey has been marked by numerous injuries and surgeries, Kevin has persevered with unwavering determination. His medical history reads like an orthopedic textbook: 6 knee operations, 2 major back surgeries, 2 hip replacements, brain surgery and brain radiation. But no amount of adversity could extinguish Kevin's inner fire and drive.

At the age of 62, Kevin undertook a monumental fitness journey to shed 60 pounds, proving that age is just a number. His passion for health and fitness remained undimmed by the passing years. Through all the ups and downs, Kevin persevered with an indomitable spirit.

He now aims to share his hard-won wisdom with others who are facing adversity. Drawing from his experiences, Kevin developed "ISO QUICK STRENGTH," a program designed to help people rebound after setbacks. He recognized that overcoming difficulties requires both physical and mental strength.

Kevin spreads his message of resilience and determination through a blog, books, and his personal mantra: "Those who quit will always fail." These simple yet powerful words encapsulate his incredible journey. After 37 remarkable years as a filmmaker, and 5 worldwide film distribution deals, Kevin now uses his gifts as a published author to share inspirational stories. With his latest release, "The Gabardine Gang," and his three best-selling books in 2024, "HYSOMETRICS," "Indie Filmmaking in the REAL WORLD," and "Hold the Power," Kevin continues to inspire and motivate readers around the world.

Earning the moniker "Life Warrior," Kevin stands as a shining example of the human capacity to overcome any adversity. His unwillingness to ever quit or back down, no matter the obstacles faced, is a testament to the motto he lives by: "A Life Warrior is willing to do whatever it takes to overcome life's challenges."

Kevin's journey has not been linear or easy. But through perseverance, inner strength, and an unbreakable warrior spirit, he has overcome obstacles that would have defeated lesser men. Though battered and bruised, Kevin stands tall as a shining example of human potential. His story is one of courage, resilience, and the power of embracing life's challenges with an open heart.

Kevin has used the visualization technique countless times. Many of his film projects were shot in his head long before filming began. During that time, Kevin has used visualization to produce Movies, TV shows, Documentaries, Music Videos and even as an Author.

Before his career in film, he was a successful powerlifter that used 'visualization' and 'positive thinking' techniques when competing. To this day, visualization is a tool Kevin uses regularly. Kevin has a motto that he lives by, "If you can see it, you can do it". After a remarkable 37-year career as a filmmaker and video producer, Kevin now wields the mighty pen to craft captivating stories in the form of books.

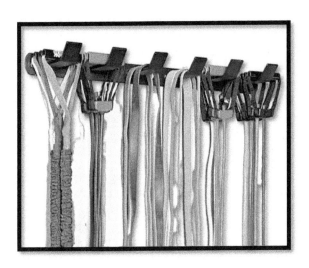

Chapter 1: Understanding the Benefits of Resistance Bands

The Versatility of Resistance Bands over weights

Resistance bands are a versatile and effective tool for strength training that can offer a wide range of benefits for individuals of all ages and fitness levels. In comparison to traditional weights, resistance bands provide a unique form of resistance that can target specific muscle groups with precision. This makes them an ideal choice for individuals looking to tone and strengthen their bodies without the need for bulky equipment or expensive gym memberships.

One of the key advantages of resistance bands over weights is their portability and convenience. Whether you are a busy teen, a working adult, or a retiree enjoying your golden years, resistance bands can easily be taken anywhere and used at any time. This means that you can fit in a quick and effective workout, regardless of where you are, whether it is at home, in the office, or on vacation.

With Resistance Bands, There Are No Excuses For Not Prioritizing Your Health And Fitness Goals.

Resistance bands offer a safer alternative to traditional weights, especially for seniors or individuals with joint issues. The controlled and gradual resistance provided by bands reduces the risk of injury, making them a suitable option for those looking to build strength without putting excessive strain on their bodies. This makes resistance bands an excellent choice for individuals recovering from injuries or looking to prevent future ones.

Furthermore, resistance bands can be easily customized to suit your individual fitness level and goals. By adjusting the tension of the band or incorporating different band exercises into your routine, you can continuously challenge your muscles and prevent plateaus in your progress. This adaptability makes resistance bands a valuable tool for individuals of all fitness levels, from beginners to advanced athletes. The versatility of resistance bands over weights makes them an essential component of any workout plan for teens, adults, and seniors alike. By incorporating resistance band exercises into your routine, you can enjoy the benefits of improved strength, flexibility, and overall fitness without the need for expensive equipment or time-consuming gym visits.

Whether you are looking to tone your body, build muscle, or simply stay active, resistance bands offer a safe, effective, and convenient solution for achieving your fitness goals.

The Importance of Strength Training for All Ages

Strength training is an essential part of any fitness routine, regardless of age. It is not just about building muscle, but also about improving overall health and well-being. For teens, adults, and seniors alike, incorporating strength training into your workout plan can have many benefits that extend beyond the gym.

Whether you are looking to increase your muscle mass, improve your bone density, or simply boost your energy levels, strength training is the key to achieving your fitness goals.

One of the most important reasons why strength training is crucial for all ages is its ability to increase muscle mass and strength. As we age, our muscle mass naturally decreases, which can lead to a decline in strength and mobility. By incorporating strength training into your workout routine, you can combat this natural process and maintain or even increase your muscle mass and strength. This is particularly essential for seniors, as it can help prevent falls and maintain independence as we age.

In addition to increasing muscle mass and strength, strength training also has numerous benefits for bone health. As we age, our bones become more fragile and prone to fractures. By engaging in regular strength training exercises, you can help maintain or even increase your bone density, reducing the risk of osteoporosis and other bone-related conditions. This is especially important for seniors, who are at a higher risk for fractures and other bone-related injuries. Furthermore, strength training can also help improve your overall health and well-being. Not only does it help to increase your metabolism and burn fat, but it can also improve your cardiovascular health, reduce your risk of chronic diseases such as diabetes and heart disease, and boost your energy levels. For teens, adults, and seniors looking to lead a healthy and active lifestyle, strength training is a crucial component of achieving and maintaining overall health.

Strength training is an essential component of any fitness routine, regardless of age. Whether you are a teen looking to increase your muscle mass, an adult looking to improve your bone density, or a senior looking to maintain your independence, incorporating strength training into your workout plan is key to achieving your fitness goals. By taking the time to prioritize strength training in your fitness routine, you can improve your muscle mass, bone density, overall health, and well-being, ensuring a happier and healthier future for yourself.

Why Resistance Bands are Ideal for Teens, Adults, and Seniors

Resistance bands are a versatile and effective tool for individuals of all ages and fitness levels. Whether you are a teen looking to stay active, an adult wanting to improve your strength and flexibility, or a senior aiming to maintain your mobility, resistance bands are the ideal choice for you. These bands offer a low-impact way to build muscle, increase endurance, and enhance overall fitness.

For teens, resistance bands provide a fun and challenging way to stay in shape. With various exercises that target different muscle groups, teens can customize their workouts to suit their individual needs and goals. Resistance bands are also portable and easy to use, making them perfect for teens with busy schedules or limited access to a gym.

Adults can benefit from resistance bands by incorporating them into their workout routines to increase strength, flexibility, and balance. Whether you are new to fitness or a seasoned athlete, resistance bands can help you achieve your fitness goals and improve your overall well-being. With consistent use, you will notice improvements in your muscle tone, posture, and overall physical performance.

Seniors can benefit from using resistance bands to maintain and improve their mobility and strength. As we age, it is important to stay active and engaged in physical activity to prevent muscle loss, improve joint health, and reduce the risk of falls. Resistance bands offer a safe and effective way for seniors to stay active and independent, allowing them to continue enjoying their favorite activities and living life to the fullest.

Resistance bands are the ideal workout tool for teens, adults, and seniors looking to improve their fitness levels and overall well-being. By incorporating resistance bands into your exercise routine, you can achieve a full-body workout that targets all major muscle groups, improves flexibility, and enhances endurance. So, grab a resistance band and get ready to unleash your full potential, no matter your age or fitness level. With dedication and consistency, you can achieve your fitness goals and live a healthier, happier life.

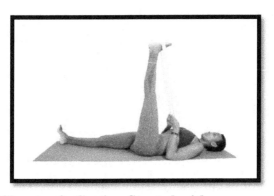

Chapter 2: Getting Started with Resistance Bands

Choosing the Right Resistance Band for Your Fitness Level

Choosing the right resistance band for your fitness level is crucial in ensuring you get the most out of your workouts. Whether you are a teen, adult, or senior, it is important to select a band that challenges you without causing strain or injury. By selecting the correct resistance band, you can tailor your workouts to your individual fitness level and gradually increase the intensity as you progress. When selecting a resistance band, consider your

current level 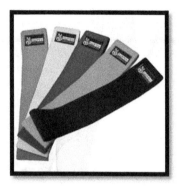 fitness and

experience with resistance training. For beginners, it is recommended to start with a light resistance band to build strength and improve muscle tone.

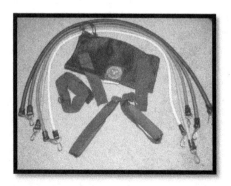

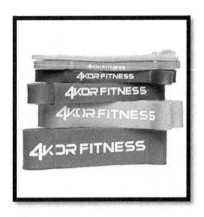

As you become more comfortable with the exercises, you can gradually increase the resistance to challenge yourself further. For more advanced individuals, a medium to heavy resistance band may be more suitable to provide the necessary intensity for a challenging workout. It is essential to listen to your body and choose a resistance band that allows you to perform each exercise with proper form and technique. Using a band that is too light will not provide enough resistance to stimulate muscle growth, while using a band that is too heavy can lead to improper form and potential injury.

By selecting the right resistance band for your fitness level, you can ensure a safe and effective workout that targets all major muscle groups.

Incorporating various resistance bands into your workout routine can help prevent plateaus and keep your muscles guessing. By alternating between light, medium, and heavy resistance bands, you can

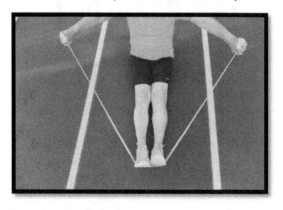

continuously challenge your muscles and prevent them from adapting to the same level of resistance.

This variety can help you achieve greater results and improve overall strength and endurance.

Remember, the key to success in fitness is consistency and dedication. By choosing the right resistance band for your fitness level and incorporating it into a comprehensive workout plan, you can achieve your health and fitness goals. With the correct mindset and determination, you can transform your body and improve your overall well-being. Select the band that challenges you, motivates you, and empowers you to become the best version of yourself.

Proper Form and Technique for Resistance Band Exercises

When it comes to resistance band exercises, proper form and technique are key to getting the most out of your workout. Whether you are a teen, adult, or senior, it is important to pay attention to your form to prevent injury and maximize the benefits of using resistance bands.

First, it is critical to pick the right resistance band for your fitness level. Bands come in assorted colors, each standing for a different level of resistance. Start with a lighter band and gradually work your way up to heavier resistance as you build strength and endurance. Remember, it's better to start off with a lighter band and work your way up than to risk injury by using a band that is too heavy for you.

Next, pay attention to your posture and alignment during resistance band exercises. Stand tall with your shoulders back and down, engaging your core muscles to support your spine. Keep your knees soft and avoid locking them out during exercises. Focus on using controlled movements and maintaining proper form throughout each exercise to target the muscles you are working.

When performing resistance band exercises, it is important to move through a full range of motion to fully engage the muscles and prevent injury. Avoid using momentum to swing the band or cheat through the exercises. Instead, focus on slow and controlled movements, pausing at the top of each exercise to squeeze the muscles before returning to the starting position. This will help you get the most out of each rep and see better results in your strength and endurance.

Listen to your body and don't push yourself beyond your limits. It's critical to challenge yourself during workouts, but it's equally essential to know when to take a break or modify an exercise if you are feeling pain or discomfort. Remember, it's better to do fewer reps with proper form than to push through with bad form and risk injury. By paying attention to your form and technique during resistance band exercises, you can safely and effectively strengthen and tone your muscles for a healthier, stronger body.

Creating a Safe and Effective Workout Space

Creating a safe and effective workout space is crucial for getting the most out of your fitness routine. Whether you are a teen, adult, or senior, it is important to set up a space that is conducive to achieving your fitness goals. By following a few simple steps, you can create a workout space that is not only safe, but also inspiring and motivating.

Primarily, it is essential to choose a space that is free from clutter and distractions. Make sure there is enough room to move freely and that you have all the equipment you need readily available. This will help you stay focused and avoid any potential hazards during your workout. Remember, safety should always be a top priority when working out, regardless of your age or fitness level.

Next, consider the lighting and ventilation in your workout space. Natural light can be energizing and uplifting, while good ventilation will help keep you cool and comfortable during your workout. If you are working out indoors, consider adding some plants or artwork to create a more welcoming and inspiring atmosphere.

Another crucial factor to consider when creating a workout space is the flooring. Make sure the floor is non-slip and provides enough cushioning to protect your joints and prevent injuries. Investing in a superior quality exercise mat can also help protect your body during floor exercises.

Finally, don't forget to personalize your workout space with items that inspire and motivate you. Whether it's a favorite quote, a picture of a loved one, or some upbeat music, adding personal touches to your workout space can help keep you motivated and on track with your fitness goals. Remember, your workout space should reflect your commitment to taking care of your body and achieving your best self.

One Single Resistance Band for an Entire Full-Body Workout

Are you looking for a simple yet effective way to get a full-body workout without the need for expensive equipment or a gym membership? Look no further than the humble resistance band. With just one single resistance band, you can target every muscle group in your body and achieve spectacular results. In this subchapter, we will explore the benefits of using a resistance band for your full-body workout and provide you with a comprehensive workout plan that is suitable for teens, adults, and seniors alike.

One of the greatest advantages of using a resistance band for your workout is its versatility. With just one band, you can perform a wide variety of exercises that target different muscle groups, including your arms, legs, chest, back, and core. This means that you can get a full-body workout without the need for multiple pieces of equipment or a complicated routine. Plus, resistance bands are lightweight and portable, making them perfect for at-home workouts or when you're on the go.

Another benefit of using a resistance band is that it helps improve your balance, stability, and flexibility. By incorporating resistance band exercises into your routine, you can strengthen your muscles in a way that mimics real-life movements, helping to prevent injury and improve your overall physical performance.

Plus, resistance bands are gentle on your joints, making them a safe and effective option for people of all ages and fitness levels. In this subchapter, we will provide you with a step-by-step workout plan that is designed to target every muscle group in your body using just one resistance band.

From bicep curls and tricep extensions to squats and lunges, we will show you how to perform each exercise with proper form and technique to maximize your results.

Whether you're a beginner looking to get started with resistance band training or a seasoned pro looking to switch up your routine, this workout plan is perfect for teens, adults, and seniors alike.

So, if you're ready to take your fitness to the next level and achieve a full-body workout with just one single resistance band, look no further than the workout plan outlined in this subchapter.

With dedication, consistency, and a positive attitude, you can transform your body and improve your overall health and well-being. Remember, it's never too late to start taking care of your body and investing in your health. Start today and see the astonishing results that you can achieve with the power of one band and one body.

Chapter 3: The Single Band Full-Body Workout Routine

Warm Up and Stretching Exercises

Welcome to the chapter on Warm Up and Stretching Exercises in "One Band, One Body: A Workout Plan for Teens, Adults & Seniors". In this section, we will discuss the importance of warming up your body before diving into your workout routine, as well as the benefits of incorporating stretching exercises into your fitness regimen.

By taking the time to thoroughly prepare your body for exercise, you can prevent injuries, improve flexibility, and enhance your overall performance.

Before you begin your workout with the single band full-body workout, it is crucial to warm up your muscles. A proper warm up increases blood flow to your muscles, making them more pliable and less susceptible to injury. Start by marching in place, doing arm circles, or performing light cardio exercises like jumping jacks or jogging in place. This will help raise your heart rate and get your body ready for the more intense exercises to come.

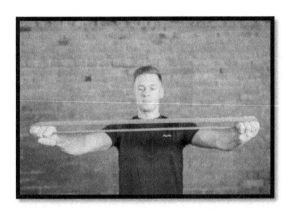

Once you have completed your warmup, it is time to move on to stretching exercises. Stretching helps improve flexibility, which can enhance your range of motion and prevent muscle tightness.

Focus on stretching the major muscle groups in your body, such as your hamstrings, quadriceps, calves, shoulders, and back. Hold each stretch for 15–30 seconds and remember to breathe deeply and relax into the stretch. Stretching should never be painful, so listen to your body and only go as far as is comfortable for you.

Incorporating warm up and stretching exercises into your workout routine is essential for maintaining good physical health and preventing injuries. By taking the time to thoroughly prepare your body for exercise, you can ensure that you can perform at your best and get the most out of your workout. Remember to listen to your body, stay hydrated, and always consult a healthcare professional before starting any new fitness regimen.

As you embark on your fitness journey with the single band full-body workout, remember to prioritize your warmup and stretching exercises. By incorporating these important steps into your routine, you can improve your flexibility, prevent injuries, and enhance your overall performance.

Stay committed to your fitness goals, stay consistent with your workouts, and always remember to take care of your body. You can achieve wonderful things – now let's get moving and make it happen!

Leg Workout

Welcome to the leg workout section of "One Band, One Body: A Workout Plan for Teens, Adults & Seniors." Whether you are a teenager looking to build strength, an adult looking to stay fit, or a senior looking to maintain mobility, this workout is designed to help you achieve your fitness goals using just one resistance band.

When it comes to working out, many people tend to focus on their upper body and neglect their lower body. However, having strong legs is essential for overall strength, balance, and mobility. This leg workout will target your quadriceps, hamstrings, glutes, and calves, helping you build muscle and improve your lower body strength.

To begin your leg workout, start with a warm-up to get your muscles ready for exercise. You can do some light cardio, such as jogging in place or jumping jacks, followed by dynamic stretches to loosen up your muscles. Once you are warmed up, grab your resistance band and get ready to work those legs!

One of the best exercises for targeting the legs with a resistance band is the squat. Stand with your feet shoulder-width apart and place the band under your feet, holding the handles at shoulder height. Lower down into a squat, keeping your chest up and back straight, then push through your heels to return to the starting position. This exercise will work your quads, hamstrings, and glutes, helping you build strength and tone your legs. Another great exercise to include in your leg workout is the leg press. Sit on the floor with your legs extended and wrap the band around the bottom of one foot, holding the handles in each hand. Press your foot against the resistance of the band, bending your knee and then straightening it to work your quads and hamstrings. Repeat on both legs to target both sides evenly. Remember to focus on proper form and control throughout each repetition to maximize the effectiveness of the exercise.

THE PROGRAM

I. Legs

In this subchapter, we will focus on one of the most important muscle groups in our body, our legs. Our legs are the foundation of our strength and mobility, allowing us to move, walk, run, and jump. By strengthening our legs, we can improve our overall fitness level and prevent injuries.

When it comes to working out our legs, there are several key exercises that can help us achieve our fitness goals. Squats, lunges, leg presses, and calf raises are all great exercises that target different muscles in our legs. By incorporating these exercises into our workout routine, we can build strength, endurance, and flexibility in our legs.

One of the best ways to work out our legs is by using resistance bands. Resistance bands are a versatile and effective tool for strengthening our muscles, including our legs.

By incorporating resistance bands into our leg workout routine, we can increase the intensity of our exercises and challenge our muscles in new ways. Remember, consistency is key when it comes to working out our legs. Make sure to set aside time each week to focus on strengthening your legs, whether it's through a full-body workout or a dedicated leg day. By staying committed to your workout routine, you will see improvements in your leg strength and overall fitness level.

Let's lace up our sneakers, grab our resistance bands, and get ready to work out our legs! Together, we can build strong and powerful legs that will support us in all our fitness endeavors. Remember,

the journey to a healthier and stronger body starts
with taking the first step — so let's start working on
our legs today!

A. Banded Squats

We will explore the benefits of incorporating
banded squats into your workout routine. Banded
squats are a fantastic exercise that targets multiple
muscle groups, including your quads, glutes, and
hamstrings.

By adding resistance with a band, you can
increase the intensity of the exercise and challenge
your muscles in new ways.

This is perfect for individuals of all fitness
levels, from teens to seniors, looking to strengthen
and tone their lower body.

One of the key advantages of banded squats is
their versatility. Whether you are a beginner or
advanced fitness enthusiast, you can adjust the
resistance of the band to suit your needs. This makes
banded squats a great exercise for teens who are just
starting their fitness journey, as well as seniors
looking to keep their strength and mobility. By
incorporating banded squats into your routine, you

can continue to progress and challenge yourself as you get stronger.

Another reason to include banded squats in your workout routine is their ability to improve functional strength. As we age, it is important to keep strong muscles to support everyday activities such as walking, climbing stairs, and bending down. Banded squats help to strengthen the muscles that are essential for these movements, making them a valuable exercise for adults and seniors looking to stay active and independent.

In addition to the physical benefits, banded squats can also have a positive impact on your mental well-being. Exercise has been shown to reduce stress, improve mood, and boost self-confidence.

By incorporating banded squats into your routine, you can experience these mental health benefits while also working towards your fitness goals. This makes banded squats a valuable tool for individuals looking to improve both their physical and mental health.

Banded squats are a fantastic exercise that can help individuals of all ages and fitness levels.

Whether you are a teen looking to build strength, an adult wanting to improve functional fitness, or a senior striving to maintain mobility, banded squats can help you achieve your goals. So, grab your band, lace up your sneakers, and get ready to squat your way to a stronger, healthier body!

B. Banded Glute Bridges

In this subchapter, we will explore the powerful exercise known as Banded Glute Bridges. This is a simple, yet effective movement is a terrific addition to your workout routine, whether you are a teen, adult, or senior looking to strengthen your lower body and improve your overall fitness. By incorporating this exercise into your workout plan, you will be on your way to achieving a stronger, more toned body.

Banded Glute Bridges are a fantastic way to target and activate your glute muscles, which are essential for stability, balance, and power in everyday activities. By using a resistance band during this exercise, you can increase the intensity and challenge your muscles even further. As you perform each rep with proper form and focus, you will feel the burn in your glutes, showing that you are effectively engaging those muscles and working towards your fitness goals.

One of the wonderful things about Banded Glute Bridges is that they can be changed to suit your individual fitness level. Whether you are a beginner just starting out or an experienced exerciser looking to push yourself to the next level, this exercise can be tailored to meet your needs. By adjusting the resistance of the band or the number of repetitions, you can customize this exercise to help you progress and see results over time.

As you incorporate Banded Glute Bridges into your workout routine, remember to focus on your form and technique to maximize the benefits of this exercise. Keep your core engaged, your back straight, and your hips lifted as you perform each rep. By keeping proper alignment and control throughout the movement, you will prevent injury and ensure that you are targeting the right muscles and getting the most out of your workout. Banded Glute Bridges are a valuable exercise that can help you strengthen your lower body, improve your overall fitness, and reach your fitness goals. Whether you are a teen, adult, or senior, this exercise can be a beneficial addition to your workout routine. Grab your resistance band, get ready to feel the burn, and start working towards a stronger, healthier you with Banded Glute Bridges.

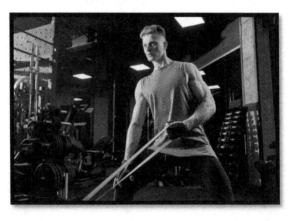

II. Back

In this section, we will focus on the importance of working out your back muscles using resistance bands. Your back is a crucial part of your body that supports your spine and helps with everyday movements. By strengthening your back muscles, you can improve your posture, reduce the risk of injury, and enhance your overall physical performance.

When it comes to working out your back with resistance bands, there are various exercises you can incorporate into your routine. From rows and pull-downs to reverse fly's and super-mans, there are plenty of options to target different areas of your back. By incorporating a mix of these exercises into your workout plan, you can ensure that you are effectively engaging all the muscles in your back.

Resistance bands are a fantastic tool for back workouts because they offer constant tension throughout the entire range of motion. This means that your muscles are continuously engaged, leading to better muscle activation and growth. Additionally, resistance bands are portable and versatile, making it easy to incorporate back exercises into your routine, regardless of where you are.

Remember, consistency is key when it comes to seeing results from your back workouts. Make sure to stay dedicated to your routine and gradually increase the resistance as you get stronger. With time and

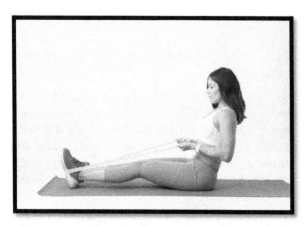

effort, you will notice improvements in your back strength, posture, and overall fitness level.

So, don't neglect your back muscles in your workout routine. By incorporating resistance band exercises into your plan, you can strengthen your back, improve your posture, and enhance your overall physical well-being. Stay motivated, stay committed, and you will see the benefits of a strong and healthy back in no time.

A. Banded Bent-Over Rows

In this subchapter, we will focus on the powerful and effective exercise known as Banded Bent-Over Rows. This exercise is a fantastic way to target multiple muscle groups in your back, shoulders, and arms, helping you build strength and definition in these key areas. By incorporating this exercise into your workout routine, you will improve your physical health and boost your confidence and overall well-being.

To perform Banded Bent-Over Rows, you will need a resistance band and a sturdy anchor point. Begin by stepping in the middle of the band with your feet shoulder-width apart and holding on to the handles with an overhand grip. Hinge at the hips, keeping your back straight and core engaged, and lower your torso until it is almost parallel to the ground. From this position, pull the band towards your lower chest, squeezing your shoulder blades together at the top of the movement. Slowly lower the band back to the starting position and repeat for a set number of repetitions.

As you perform Banded Bent-Over Rows, focus on keeping proper form and controlled movements. This exercise requires both strength and stability, so be sure to engage your core and keep your back straight throughout each repetition. By challenging yourself with a resistance band, you will build muscle and improve your balance and coordination, leading to better overall functional fitness. Incorporating

Banded Bent-Over Rows into your workout routine will help you develop a strong and toned upper body, enhancing your posture and overall physical appearance. This exercise is a fantastic way to target key muscle groups that are often neglected in traditional workouts, making it a valuable addition to any fitness regimen. By committing to regular practice and gradually increasing the resistance of the band, you will see improvements in your strength, endurance, and overall fitness level.

Remember, consistency is key when it comes to achieving your fitness goals. By incorporating Banded Bent-Over Rows into your regular workout routine, you are taking a proactive step towards improving your physical health and well-being. Embrace the challenge, stay motivated, and push yourself to new heights with this powerful exercise. You have the strength and determination to succeed, so keep pushing forward and watch as your body transforms before your eyes.

B. Banded Lat Pulldowns

In this subchapter, we will explore the benefits of banded lat pulldowns, a powerful exercise that targets the muscles of the back and arms. Whether you are a teen, adult, or senior, incorporating banded lat pulldowns into your workout routine can help improve your strength, posture, and overall fitness level.

This exercise is especially beneficial for individuals following "The Single Band Full-Body Workout" plan, as it provides a challenging yet effective way to work multiple muscle groups with just one simple piece of equipment. Banded lat pulldowns are a versatile exercise that can be adapted to suit your individual fitness level. By adjusting the tension of the band, you can make the exercise easier or more challenging to match your strength and abilities. This makes it an ideal choice for beginners who are just starting their fitness journey, as well as seasoned gym-goers looking to push themselves to new heights. No matter where you are on your fitness journey, banded lat pulldowns can help you reach your goals and achieve the results you wish.

One of the key benefits of banded lat pulldowns is their ability to target the lats, or latissimus dorsi muscles, which are the largest muscles in the back. By strengthening these muscles, you can improve your posture, reduce the risk of injury, and enhance your overall athletic performance. Additionally, banded lat pulldowns engage the muscles of the arms, shoulders, and core, providing a full-body workout that can help you build strength and endurance in multiple areas. With consistent practice and dedication, banded lat pulldowns can help you achieve a toned, sculpted physique that will leave you feeling strong and confident.

As you incorporate banded lat pulldowns into your workout routine, remember to focus on proper form and technique to maximize the benefits of the exercise. Keep your back straight, shoulders down and back, and engage your core muscles to support your spine throughout the movement. Exhale as you pull the band down towards your chest, and inhale as you return to the starting position.

By paying attention to these details and listening to your body, you can ensure that you are performing banded lat pulldowns safely and effectively and getting the most out of your workout. Banded lat pulldowns are a valuable addition to any workout routine, offering a multitude of benefits for individuals of all ages and fitness levels. By incorporating this exercise into "The Single Band

Full-Body Workout" plan, you can strengthen your back, arms, and core, improve your posture, and enhance your overall fitness level.

With dedication, consistency, and a positive attitude, banded lat pulldowns can help you achieve your fitness goals and become the best version of yourself. Get ready to work hard and watch as your strength and confidence soar to new heights with banded lat pulldowns.

III. Chest

We focus on the chest muscles and how to effectively target them using resistance bands. The chest muscles are an essential part of our upper body strength and play a crucial role in many everyday activities. By incorporating chest exercises into your workout routine, you can improve your overall strength and posture.

When working out the chest muscles, it is important to use proper form to prevent injury and maximize results. Start by anchoring your resistance band securely to a door frame or another stable surface. Stand facing away from the anchor point and grasp the handles of the resistance band with your hands at chest level. As you push forward, focus on squeezing your chest muscles and keeping a controlled movement.

One effective exercise for targeting the chest muscles is the chest press. This exercise mimics the motion of a bench press but uses resistance bands instead of weights. To perform a chest press, sit on a stability ball or chair with your feet firmly planted on the ground. Hold the resistance band handles at chest level and push forward until your arms are fully extended. Slowly return to the starting position and repeat for a set number of repetitions.

Another great chest exercise to incorporate into your workout routine is the chest fly. This exercise targets the chest muscles from a different angle and helps to improve overall muscle balance. To perform a chest fly, lie on your back on a mat with your knees bent and feet flat on the floor. Hold the resistance band handles above your chest with your arms slightly bent. Slowly open your arms out to the sides, keeping a slight bend in your elbows, then return to the starting position.

Remember to listen to your body and adjust the resistance level of the band as needed. As you continue to challenge yourself and push your limits, you will see improvements in your chest strength and overall fitness. Stay focused, stay motivated, and keep pushing yourself to reach your fitness goals. Your chest muscles will thank you for the demanding work you put in.

A. Banded Push-Ups

We will explore the benefits of incorporating banded push-ups into your workout routine. Banded push-ups are a terrific way to challenge your upper body strength and target multiple muscle groups. By using a resistance band, you can increase the intensity of this classic exercise and take your workout to the next level.

To perform banded push-ups, start by securing the resistance band around your back and holding on to the ends with your hands. As you lower yourself down into a push-up position, the band will provide added resistance, forcing your muscles to work harder. This increased resistance helps to build strength in your chest, shoulders, and triceps, making banded push-ups a fantastic exercise for anyone looking to improve their upper body strength.

One of the key benefits of banded push-ups is that they can be easily changed to suit your fitness level. Whether you are a beginner or an experienced athlete, you can adjust the tension of the resistance band to increase or decrease the difficulty of the exercise. This versatility makes banded push-ups an excellent choice for teens, adults, and seniors alike, as everyone can tailor the exercise to their individual needs.

In addition to building strength, banded push-ups also help to improve your stability and balance. By engaging your core muscles to control the resistance of the band, you are working your upper body and strengthening your core. This added stability can help to prevent injuries and improve your overall performance in other exercises and daily activities. So, if you're looking to challenge yourself and take your workout to the next level, give banded push-ups a try. Incorporating this exercise into your routine will help you build strength, improve stability, and enhance your overall fitness level. Remember, with dedication and consistency, you can achieve your fitness goals and become the best version of yourself.

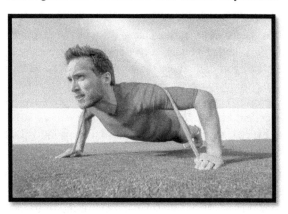

B. Banded Chest Press

The benefits of the Banded Chest Press, a powerful exercise that can help you strengthen and tone your chest muscles.

This exercise is perfect for individuals of all ages, whether you are a teen looking to build muscle, an adult striving for a healthier lifestyle, or a senior wanting to maintain strength and mobility. The Banded Chest Press is a versatile exercise that can be easily modified to suit your fitness level, making it a fantastic addition to your workout routine.

When performing the Banded Chest Press, it is important to focus on proper form and technique. Start by lying on your back with your knees bent and feet flat on the floor. Hold the resistance band at chest level with your palms facing away from you. Slowly press the band away from your body until your arms are fully extended, then return to the starting position. Remember to engage your core throughout the exercise to stabilize your body and prevent injury.

One of the key benefits of the Banded Chest Press is its ability to target the chest muscles, including the pectoralis major and minor. By incorporating this exercise into your workout routine, you can improve your upper body strength and definition. Additionally, the Banded Chest Press can help improve your posture and reduce the risk of shoulder injuries by strengthening the muscles that support the shoulder joint. With consistent practice, you will notice an increase in your overall upper body strength and endurance.

As you continue to perform the Banded Chest Press, challenge yourself by increasing the resistance of the band or incorporating different variations of the exercise. Whether you are a beginner or an experienced fitness enthusiast, there are endless ways to customize this exercise to suit your individual needs and goals. Remember to listen to your body and adjust as needed to ensure a safe and effective workout. With dedication and perseverance, you will see progress and improvement in your strength and fitness levels.

The Banded Chest Press is a valuable exercise that can help individuals of all ages and fitness levels. By incorporating this exercise into your workout routine, you can strengthen and tone your chest muscles, improve your posture, and reduce the risk of shoulder injuries. Remember to focus on proper form and technique, challenge yourself by increasing the resistance, and listen to your body to ensure a safe and effective workout. With dedication and consistency, you can achieve your fitness goals and transform your body with the power of the Banded Chest Press.

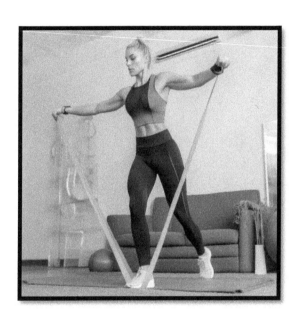

IV. Shoulders

Here, we will focus on the often neglected but crucial part of our bodies — the shoulders. Our shoulders play a vital role in our everyday movements, from reaching for items on high shelves to throwing a ball or even just giving someone a hug. By strengthening our shoulders, we can improve our overall fitness and prevent injuries.

To begin, let's discuss the importance of shoulder exercises in our workout routine. Strong shoulders are essential for maintaining good posture, preventing shoulder injuries, and enhancing our overall athletic performance. By incorporating shoulder exercises into our workout plan, we can build strength and stability in this area, leading to improved function and mobility. One of the most effective ways to strengthen our shoulders is through resistance band exercises. By using a resistance band, we can target specific muscles in the shoulders and work on improving their strength and endurance.

Whether you are a teen, adult, or senior, resistance band exercises are a safe and effective way to build shoulder strength without the need for heavy weights or expensive equipment.

Incorporating shoulder exercises into our workout routine can also have a positive impact on our mental wellbeing. Strong shoulders can improve our confidence and self-esteem, as well as reduce stress and anxiety. By taking care of our bodies and prioritizing our physical health, we can enhance our overall sense of wellbeing and lead a more fulfilling life. Don't overlook the importance of shoulder exercises in your workout routine. By strengthening your shoulders with resistance band exercises, you can improve your posture, prevent injuries, and enhance your overall fitness. Remember, our bodies are all connected, and by taking care of our shoulders, we are taking care of our entire body. Start working on those shoulders today!

A. Banded Lateral Raises

Welcome to the subchapter on Banded Lateral Raises in our book "One Band, One Body: A Workout Plan for Teens, Adults & Seniors." This exercise is perfect for individuals of all ages and fitness levels who are looking to strengthen their shoulders and improve their overall muscle tone. By incorporating banded lateral raises into your workout routine, you will see physical results and gain confidence and a sense of accomplishment.

To perform banded lateral raises, simply stand with your feet shoulder-width apart, holding on to the band with both hands. Keep a slight bend in your elbows and raise your arms out to the sides until they are parallel to the floor. Slowly lower them back down to the starting position and repeat for a set number of repetitions. This exercise targets the deltoid muscles in your shoulders, helping to build strength and definition.

As you continue to practice banded lateral raises, you will notice an improvement in your posture and overall upper body strength. Your shoulders will become more defined, giving you a toned and sculpted appearance. This exercise is also great for improving shoulder stability and reducing the risk of injury during other workouts or daily activities.

Incorporating banded lateral raises into your workout routine will not only help you physically but also mentally. As you challenge yourself to complete each repetition, you will build resilience and determination. The sense of accomplishment that comes from mastering this exercise will boost your self-confidence and motivate you to continue pushing yourself in other areas of your life. Remember, consistency is key when it comes to seeing results from your workouts. Make banded lateral raises a regular part of your exercise routine and watch as your strength and muscle tone improve over time. Stay motivated, stay dedicated, and most importantly, have fun with your workouts.

You can achieve important things, and banded lateral raises are just the beginning of your fitness journey.

B. Banded Front Raises

We look at the Banded Front Raises, a powerful exercise that targets your shoulder muscles and helps improve your overall upper body strength. This exercise is perfect for teens, adults, and seniors looking to tone and define their shoulders while also improving their posture and stability.

By incorporating Banded Front Raises into your workout routine, you can challenge yourself and push your limits to achieve the results you want.

To perform Banded Front Raises, start by standing with your feet shoulder-width apart and holding the resistance band in both hands. Keep your arms straight and slowly raise them in front of you, making sure to engage your shoulder muscles throughout the movement. Focus on keeping a controlled and steady pace to maximize the effectiveness of this exercise. As you raise your arms, visualize yourself becoming stronger and more confident with each repetition.

As you continue to perform Banded Front Raises, you will feel your shoulder muscles working hard and getting stronger with each set. Embrace the burn and push through any discomfort, knowing that you are on your way to achieving your fitness goals. Remember that consistency is key, so make sure to include this exercise in your regular workout routine to see progress and improvements over time.

Stay dedicated and motivated, and you will soon reap the rewards of your hard work and determination. Incorporating Banded Front Raises into your workout routine is not just about physical strength, but also about mental strength and resilience. Use this exercise as an opportunity to challenge yourself and push past any self-imposed limitations. Believe in your ability to achieve greatness, and let that belief drive you towards success. With dedication and perseverance, you can conquer any obstacle and become the best version of yourself. As you conclude your Banded Front Raises workout, take a moment to reflect on the progress you have made and the obstacles you have overcome. Celebrate your achievements, no matter how small they may seem, and use them as fuel to keep pushing forward. Remember that you can achieve anything you set your mind to, and with the power of Banded Front Raises and your unwavering determination, there is no limit to what you can carry out. Keep up the magnificent work, stay motivated, and continue to strive for greatness in all aspects of your life.

V. Triceps

In this chapter, we will focus on the powerful and often overlooked muscle group known as the triceps. The triceps are found on the back of your upper arms and are essential for everyday movements such as pushing, pulling, and lifting.

By strengthening your triceps, you can improve your overall arm strength and enhance your performance in various exercises and activities. To effectively target your triceps, we will introduce you to a series of exercises using just one resistance band. This versatile piece of equipment is all you need to engage your triceps and unlock their full potential. With the right technique and consistency, you will see noticeable improvements in your arm strength and muscle tone.

One of the key benefits of training your triceps is the impact it can have on your overall physique. Strong and defined triceps contribute to a more sculpted appearance and improve your posture and stability. By incorporating triceps exercises into your workout routine, you will enhance your physical appearance and boost your confidence and self-esteem.

Whether you are a teen looking to build strength, an adult looking to stay active, or a senior wanting to keep independence, strengthening your triceps is crucial for overall health and well-being. By dedicating time and effort to your triceps workouts, you are investing in a stronger, more resilient body that will serve you well in all aspects of your life. So, grab your resistance band and get ready to unlock the full potential of your triceps on your journey to a healthier and happier you.

A. Banded Triceps Pushdowns

Are you looking to strengthen and sculpt your triceps? Look no further than banded triceps pushdowns! This exercise is a fantastic way to target and tone your triceps, helping you achieve the strong and defined arms you desire. In this subchapter, we will explore the benefits of banded triceps pushdowns and provide you with a step-by-step guide on how to perform this exercise effectively.

Banded triceps pushdowns are a powerful addition to your workout routine because they specifically target the triceps, which can often be a challenging area to tone. By using a resistance band, you can adjust the level of resistance to suit your fitness level, making this exercise accessible for teens, adults, and seniors alike. With consistent practice, banded triceps pushdowns can help you build strength and endurance in your triceps, leading to improved overall arm strength. To perform banded triceps pushdowns, start by attaching a resistance band to a sturdy overhead structure, such as a pull-up bar or door frame. Stand facing the band with your feet shoulder-width apart and grasp the band with an overhand grip. Keeping your elbows close to your sides, extend your arms downward, engaging your triceps as you push the band toward the ground. Slowly return to the starting position and repeat for a set number of repetitions.

As you practice banded triceps pushdowns, remember to focus on your form and technique to ensure you are targeting the triceps effectively. Keep your core engaged and maintain a strong posture throughout the exercise to maximize the benefits for your triceps. With dedication and perseverance, banded triceps pushdowns can help you achieve the toned and sculpted arms you want. Incorporate banded triceps pushdowns into your regular workout routine to experience the transformative power of this exercise.

As you challenge yourself and push your limits, you will strengthen your triceps and build confidence in your abilities. Embrace the journey of self-improvement and let banded tricep pushdowns be a cornerstone of your fitness journey towards a stronger, healthier you.

B. Banded Overhead Tricep Extensions

Welcome to the subchapter on Banded Overhead Tricep Extensions. This exercise is a fantastic way to target and strengthen your triceps using just one resistance band. Whether you are a teen looking to build muscle, an adult looking to tone your arms, or a senior wanting to improve your upper body strength, this exercise is perfect for all fitness levels.

To perform Banded Overhead Tricep Extensions, start by standing in the middle of the resistance band with your feet hip-width apart. Hold one end of the band in each hand, bringing your arms overhead with your elbows bent and close to your ears. Slowly extend your arms straight up towards the ceiling, feeling the resistance in your triceps.

Lower your arms back down to the starting position and repeat for a set of 12–15 reps. Remember, proper form is key when performing Banded Overhead Tricep Extensions. Keep your core engaged, your back straight, and your elbows close to your ears throughout the movement. Focus on the mind-muscle connection, feeling the burn in your triceps with each repetition. Take your time and listen to your body, adjusting the resistance as needed to challenge yourself while keeping proper form. As you incorporate Banded Overhead Tricep Extensions into your workout routine, you will begin to see improvements in your arm strength and muscle definition. Consistency is key, so aim to perform this exercise 2–3 times a week to see the best results. Remember, progress takes time, so be patient with yourself and celebrate every small victory along the way.

Banded Overhead Tricep Extensions are a powerful exercise that can help you achieve your fitness goals and strengthen your upper body. Whether you are a teen, adult, or senior, this exercise is a great addition to your workout routine. Keep pushing yourself, stay motivated, and most importantly, have fun with your fitness journey. You can achieve anything you set your mind to, so let's crush those tricep extensions and continue to work towards a stronger, healthier you!

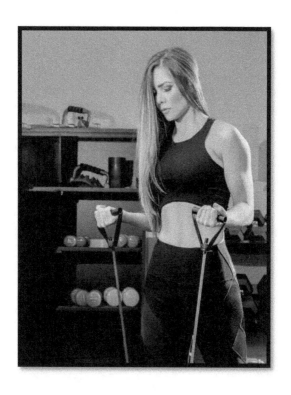

VI. Biceps

Welcome to Chapter VI of "One Band, One Body: A Workout Plan for Teens, Adults & Seniors" where we will be focusing on strengthening and toning one of the most iconic muscles in the body — the biceps. Whether you are a teen looking to build confidence, an adult aiming for a more sculpted physique, or a senior seeking to support strength and mobility, this chapter is for you.

The biceps are not only a symbol of strength and power, but they also play a crucial role in everyday movements such as lifting groceries, carrying bags, and even just picking up your child or grandchild. By targeting and training this muscle group, you can improve your overall functional fitness and enhance your quality of life.

Here, we will be exploring various exercises using just one resistance band to effectively target and strengthen your biceps.

From bicep curls to hammer curls to concentration curls, you will learn how to execute each movement properly with precision and control to maximize muscle engagement and growth.

As you embark on this journey to sculpt and strengthen your biceps, remember that consistency is key. By incorporating these exercises into your regular workout routine and gradually increasing the resistance level of your band as you progress, you will see improvements in both the size and strength of your biceps over time.

So, grab your resistance band, harness your determination, and get ready to feel the burn as you work towards building the biceps of your dreams. With dedication, persistence, and a positive mindset, you can achieve your fitness goals and become the best version of yourself. Let's flex those muscles and show the world what you're made of!

A. Banded Bicep Curls

We explore the benefits and techniques of one of the most effective exercises you can do with a resistance band — Banded Bicep Curls. This exercise is perfect for teens, adults, and seniors looking to tone and strengthen their arms, as well as improve their overall fitness levels. By incorporating Banded

Bicep Curls into your workout routine, you will not only see physical improvements, but you will also feel more confident and empowered in your body.

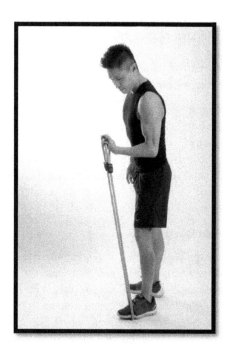

Banded Bicep Curls target the biceps, which are the muscles on the front of your upper arms. By performing this exercise regularly, you can sculpt and define your biceps, giving you strong and toned arms. Whether you are looking to increase your muscle mass or simply improve your arm strength, Banded Bicep Curls are a fantastic choice for achieving your fitness goals. With just a resistance band and a positive attitude, you can transform your arms and build the strength you desire.

To perform Banded Bicep Curls, start by standing with your feet hip-width apart and placing the resistance band under both feet. Hold the handles of the band with an underhand grip, palms facing up. Keeping your elbows close to your sides, slowly curl your hands towards your shoulders, squeezing your biceps at the top of the movement. Slowly lower your hands back down to the starting position, maintain control throughout the exercise.

Aim for 3 sets of 12–15 reps, focusing on proper form and engaging your biceps with each repetition.

As you incorporate Banded Bicep Curls into your workout routine, remember to challenge yourself and push beyond your limits. With dedication and perseverance, you can achieve incredible results and transform your body.

By focusing on the mind-muscle connection and keeping proper form, you will maximize the benefits of this exercise and see real progress in your arm strength and definition. Stay committed to your fitness journey and believe in the power of your body to change and grow stronger with each workout.

Banded Bicep Curls are a fantastic addition to your fitness routine, no matter your age or fitness level. By incorporating this exercise into your workout plan, you can sculpt and strengthen your arms, boost your confidence, and improve your overall health and well-being. Remember to stay consistent, push yourself to new heights, and embrace the journey of self-improvement. With the power of one band and one body, you can achieve your fitness goals and unlock your full potential.

B. Banded Hammer Curls

The banded hammer curls — an incredible exercise that targets the biceps and forearms. This exercise is perfect for individuals of all ages, whether you are a teen looking to build strength, an adult striving for a more toned physique, or a senior wanting to keep muscle mass and mobility. By incorporating banded hammer curls into your workout routine, you will sculpt your arms and improve your overall strength and functionality.

Banded hammer curls are a versatile exercise that can be performed anywhere with just a single resistance band. This makes them perfect for those who prefer to work out at home or on the go.

The controlled movement of the hammer curl targets the biceps and forearms, helping to build muscle and increase strength in these areas. By incorporating this exercise into your routine, you will notice an increase in your arm definition and overall upper body strength.

One of the great benefits of banded hammer curls is their ability to engage multiple muscle groups simultaneously. By maintaining proper form and focusing on the contraction of the biceps and forearms, you will also engage your core and stabilizer muscles. This helps to improve your overall strength and enhances your balance and coordination.

As you continue to incorporate banded hammer curls into your workout routine, you will notice improvements in your overall fitness and functionality.

As you progress in your fitness journey, you may choose to increase the resistance of the band to challenge yourself further. This will help to continue to build muscle and strength in your arms, allowing you to reach new levels of fitness and performance.

Remember to always listen to your body and adjust the resistance as needed to ensure you are working at a level that is challenging yet achievable.

With dedication and consistency, you will see progress and improvements in your strength and physique. Banded hammer curls are a fantastic exercise that can help individuals of all ages and fitness levels. Whether you are a teen, adult, or senior, incorporating this exercise into your workout routine will help you achieve your fitness goals and improve your overall strength and functionality. Get ready to sculpt your arms and build muscle with banded hammer curls. Remember, consistency is key, and with dedication and hard work, you can achieve the results you are looking for.

Core Strengthening Exercises with Resistance Bands

Welcome to the subchapter on core strengthening exercises with resistance bands in "One Band, One Body: A Workout Plan for Teens, Adults & Seniors." In this section, we will explore how you can use a simple resistance band to target and strengthen your core muscles, helping you build a solid foundation for all your other physical activities.

Core strength is essential for proper posture, preventing back pain, and improving overall stability and balance. By incorporating resistance bands into your core workouts, you can add an extra challenge that will help you develop a strong and stable core. These exercises are suitable for teens, adults, and seniors of all fitness levels, get your band and get ready to feel the burn!

One of the best core strengthening exercises you can do with a resistance band is the standing oblique twist. Simply hold one end of the resistance band in each hand, extend your arms in front of you, and twist your torso from side to side, engaging your oblique muscles. This exercise targets your core and helps improve your balance and coordination.

Another effective core exercise with resistance bands is the plank row. Start in a plank position with the resistance band looped around your wrists. Keep your body in a straight line from head to heels as you alternate rowing each arm back, engaging your core muscles to stabilize your body.

This Exercise Strengthens your Core and Works your Shoulders, Back, and Arms.

As you continue to incorporate core-strengthening exercises with resistance bands into your workout routine, remember to focus on proper form and technique. Engage your core muscles throughout each movement and listen to your body to avoid overexertion or injury.

With consistent practice and dedication, you will build a strong and stable core that will support you in all your physical activities and improve your overall health and well-being. Grab your band, get moving, and feel the transformation in your core strength!

Chapter 4: Progressing Your Workouts with Resistance Bands

Increasing Resistance and Intensity Safely

To see continuous progress in your fitness journey, it is important to increase resistance and intensity safely. This will not only challenge your body in new ways, but also help you build strength and endurance over time. As we age, it becomes even more crucial to push ourselves out of our comfort zones and take our workouts to the next level.

One way to safely increase resistance is by using a heavier resistance band. As you become stronger, you may find that the band you started with no longer provides enough of a challenge. Gradually increasing the resistance will help you continue to see improvements in your strength and muscle tone. Remember, it's important to listen to your body and not push yourself too hard too quickly. Slow and steady progress is key.

Another way to ramp up the intensity of your workouts is by increasing the number of sets and reps you do. By adding an extra set or increasing the number of repetitions, you can push your muscles to work harder and grow stronger.

This can help you break through plateaus and see continued progress in your fitness goals. Just be sure to maintain proper form throughout your workout to prevent injury.

Incorporating high-intensity interval training (HIIT) into your workout routine is another effective way to increase resistance and intensity safely. HIIT involves short bursts of intense exercise followed by periods of rest or lower-intensity exercise.

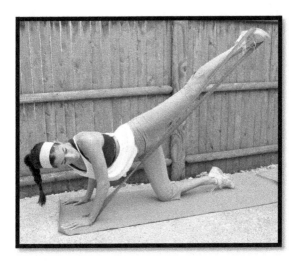

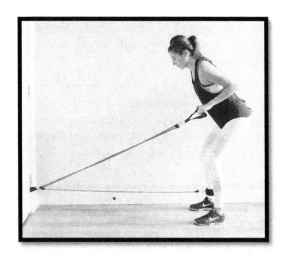

This type of workout not only challenges your cardiovascular system, but also helps build strength and endurance. Just be sure to start slow and gradually increase the intensity as you become more comfortable with the exercises. Remember, the key to increasing resistance and intensity safely is to listen to your body and adjust as needed. Push yourself out of your comfort zone, but also know your limits. By gradually increasing resistance, adding sets and reps, and incorporating HIIT into your routine, you can continue to see improvements in your strength, endurance, and overall fitness levels. Stay motivated, stay consistent, and keep pushing yourself to be the best version of yourself.

Incorporating Cardiovascular Exercises with Resistance Bands

Incorporating cardiovascular exercises with resistance bands can take your workout to the next level and help you achieve your fitness goals faster. By combining the benefits of both types of exercise, you can improve your cardiovascular health, build strength and endurance, and increase your overall fitness level. In this subchapter, we will explore how to effectively incorporate cardiovascular exercises with resistance bands into your workout routine.

Cardiovascular exercises, such as running, cycling, and jumping jacks, are great for increasing your heart rate and improving your endurance. When combined with resistance bands, these exercises become even more challenging and effective. By adding resistance bands to your cardio routine, you can engage multiple muscle groups at once, leading to a more intense and efficient workout. This combination of cardiovascular and strength training will help you burn more calories, build lean muscle, and improve your overall fitness level. One of the best ways to incorporate cardiovascular exercises with resistance bands is to perform circuit training. Circuit training involves performing a series of exercises back-to-back with minimal rest in between.

By alternating between cardiovascular exercises and resistance band exercises, you can keep your heart rate elevated while also challenging your muscles in separate ways. This type of workout is not only effective for burning calories and building strength, but it also keeps your workouts interesting and engaging.

Another way to incorporate cardiovascular exercises with resistance bands is to include interval training in your routine. Interval training involves alternating between high-intensity bursts of exercise and periods of rest or low-intensity activity. By using resistance bands during your high-intensity intervals, you can increase the intensity of your workout and push your muscles to work harder. This type of training is great for improving cardiovascular fitness, burning fat, and building lean muscle mass.

Incorporating cardiovascular exercises with resistance bands is a great way to challenge your body, improve your fitness level, and achieve your health and wellness goals. Whether you are a teen, adult, or senior, adding resistance bands to your cardio routine can help you take your workouts to the next level and see faster results. Lace up your sneakers and get ready to elevate your workout with this powerful combination of exercises.

Tracking Your Progress and Setting Goals

Congratulations on taking the first step towards improving your health and fitness with the Single Band Full-Body Workout plan! As you embark on this journey, it is important to track your progress and set goals to keep yourself motivated and on track. By checking your improvements and setting achievable goals, you will stay focused and committed to reaching your ultimate fitness goals. One of the best ways to track your progress is by keeping a workout journal. Write down the exercises you do, the number

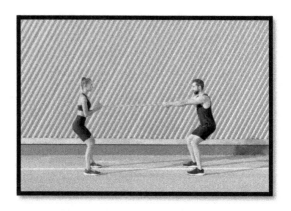

of repetitions and sets, and any modifications you make to the workouts.

You can also track your weight, measurements, and how you feel after each workout. Seeing your progress written down can be incredibly motivating and help you stay accountable to yourself.

In addition to tracking your progress, it is essential to set specific, measurable, achievable, relevant, and time-bound (SMART) goals. Whether your goal is to lose weight, build muscle, or improve your overall fitness level, having a clear goal in mind will keep you focused and driven. Break down your goal into smaller, more manageable milestones that you can work towards each week or month.

Remember, progress is not always linear, and setbacks are a natural part of any fitness journey. If you experience a setback, don't get discouraged. Instead, reflect on what may have caused the setback and use it as an opportunity to learn and grow.

Adjust your goals if needed and keep pushing forward. You can achieve anything you set your mind to with dedication and perseverance.

Tracking your progress and setting goals are crucial components of any successful fitness plan. By watching your improvements, setting SMART goals, and staying resilient in the face of setbacks, you will be well on your way to achieving your fitness goals.

Remember, you can do this! Stay focused, stay motivated, and keep pushing yourself to be the best version of yourself.

Chapter 5: Staying Motivated and Consistent with Your Workout

Finding Your "Why" for Working Out

Finding your "why" for working out. It is essential staying motivated and committed to your fitness journey. Understanding the reasons behind why you want to improve your physical health can help you push through the tough days and stay focused on your goals. Whether you are a teen, adult, or senior, having a strong "why" can make all the difference in your workout routine.

For teens, finding your "why" for working out could be as simple as wanting to feel more confident in your skin or improving your athletic performance. You have a goal of making the varsity team next season, or you simply want to have more energy throughout the day. Whatever your reason may be, showing your "why" can help you stay dedicated to your fitness routine and see the results you desire.

Adults often have assorted reasons for working out, whether it be to manage stress, improve overall health, or maintain a healthy weight. Finding your "why" can help you stay consistent with your workouts, even when life gets busy. You want to set a positive example for your children, or you have a specific fitness goal in mind, such as running a marathon or completing a triathlon. Whatever your motivation may be, keeping your "why" at the forefront of your mind can help you stay on track and reach your fitness goals.

Seniors may have several reasons for working out, such as improving mobility, keeping independence, or preventing age-related health issues. Finding your "why" can help you stay active

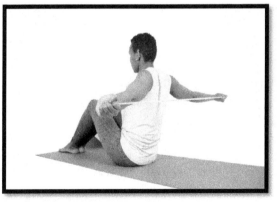

and healthy as you age, allowing you to enjoy a

higher quality of life. Whether you want to stay strong and mobile to keep up with your grandchildren or you simply would like to feel better in your body, having a strong "why" can keep you motivated to stay consistent with your workouts.

No matter your age or fitness level, naming your "why" for working out is crucial in staying motivated and committed to your fitness routine. Whether you are a teen, adult, or senior, finding your motivation can help you push through the tough days and stay focused on your goals. Take some time to reflect on why you want to improve your physical health and use that as fuel to drive your workouts. Remember, your "why" is unique to you and can be a powerful tool in achieving your fitness goals.

Overcoming Challenges and Setbacks

Life is full of challenges and setbacks, but it is how we choose to overcome them that truly defines us. In the realm of fitness, setbacks can come in many forms from injuries to plateaus in progress. However, it is important to remember that with determination and perseverance, anything is possible. As we embark on our fitness journey with the Single Band Full-Body Workout, let us embrace the challenges that come our way and use them as opportunities for growth and self-improvement.

One of the keyways to overcome challenges and setbacks in our fitness journey is to stay focused on our goals. It can be easy to get discouraged when faced with obstacles, but by keeping our eyes on the prize and reminding ourselves of why we started this journey in the first place, we can find the strength to push through. Whether your goal is to lose weight, gain muscle, or simply improve your overall health, staying focused and determined will help you overcome any obstacle that comes your way.

Another important aspect of overcoming challenges and setbacks is to be adaptable and flexible in our approach. Occasionally, the best-laid plans can go awry, and it is important to be able to pivot and adjust our strategies as needed. If an injury prevents us from doing a certain exercise, we can find alternative ways to work those muscles. If we hit a plateau in our progress, we can switch up our routine to keep our bodies guessing. By staying adaptable and open-minded, we can overcome any obstacle that comes our way. In addition to staying focused and adaptable, it is also important to seek support and encouragement from others.

Whether it be friends, family, or a workout buddy, having a support system can make all the difference when facing challenges in our fitness journey. Surrounding ourselves with positive and like-minded individuals can provide us with the motivation and inspiration we need to keep pushing forward, even when the going gets tough. The key to overcoming challenges and setbacks in our fitness journey is to never give up. No matter how difficult the road may seem, remember that every setback is just a steppingstone on the path to success. By staying focused on our goals, being adaptable in our approach, seeking support from others, and never giving up, we can conquer any obstacle that comes our way. So let us embrace the challenges that come our way with determination and perseverance, knowing that we can achieve anything we set our minds to.

Celebrating Your Achievements and Progress

Congratulations on completing another successful workout session! It's important to take a moment to celebrate your achievements and progress along your fitness journey. Whether you are a teen, an adult, or a senior, each step you take towards improving your health and well-being is worth recognizing and celebrating. Remember, every small victory brings you closer to your ultimate fitness goals. Reflect on how far you have come since starting the Single Band Full-Body Workout plan. Have you noticed improvements in your strength, endurance, or flexibility? Maybe you can now perform an exercise that was once challenging for you, or you have increased the intensity of your workouts.

Take pride in these accomplishments and give yourself a well-deserved pat on the back. Don't forget to acknowledge the hard work and dedication that you have put into your fitness routine. It takes commitment and perseverance to stick to a workout plan, especially when faced with obstacles or setbacks. Your willingness to show up and push yourself each day is a testament to your strength and determination. Keep up the great work and remember that every effort you put in brings you closer to reaching your fitness goals. As you celebrate your achievements and progress, take a moment to set new goals for yourself. Whether it's increasing the number of reps or sets in your workout, trying a new exercise, or improving your overall fitness level, having clear goals can help keep you motivated and focused. Remember, consistency is key, and by continuing to challenge yourself, you will continue to see progress and improvements in your fitness journey.

Take the time to celebrate your achievements and progress along your fitness journey. Embrace the challenges, setbacks, and victories that come with each workout session, and use them as fuel to keep pushing yourself towards your goals. Remember, with dedication, determination, and a positive attitude, you can reach new heights in your fitness journey. Keep up the wonderful work, and never underestimate the power of celebrating your successes along the way.

Chapter 6: The Mind-Body Connection in Fitness

The Role of Mental Health in Physical Wellbeing

It is crucial to recognize the interconnectedness of mental health and physical wellbeing when it comes to achieving overall health and wellness. In our journey towards fitness and strength, we must not overlook the power of our minds in shaping our bodies. The way we perceive ourselves, our thoughts and emotions, all play a significant role in our physical health. When we prioritize our mental health, we are laying a durable foundation for our physical wellbeing.

As we engage in the Single Band Full-Body Workout, it is important to remember that our mental state can impact our physical performance. When we approach our workouts with a positive mindset, we are more likely to push ourselves to new limits and achieve our fitness goals.

On the contrary, negative thoughts and self-doubt can hinder our progress and limit our potential. By cultivating a positive attitude and practicing self-care, we can enhance our physical capabilities and improve our workout results. Mindfulness and stress management are key components of mental health that can significantly affect our physical wellbeing. Incorporating relaxation techniques such as deep breathing, meditation, and yoga into our workout routine can help reduce stress levels and improve our overall health.

By taking the time to focus on our mental wellbeing, we are creating a harmonious balance between mind and body, leading to better physical outcomes and a more fulfilling fitness journey. In times of challenges and setbacks, it is important to prioritize our mental health to maintain our physical wellbeing.

By practicing resilience and perseverance, we can overcome obstacles and continue to progress towards our fitness goals. Remember that setbacks are a natural part of the journey, and by approaching them with a positive mindset, we can learn and grow stronger. Embrace the power of your mind in shaping your body, and trust in your ability to achieve greatness through the Single Band Full-Body Workout.

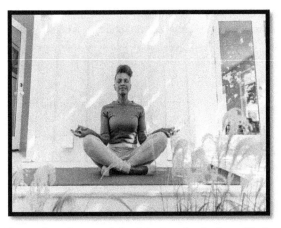

The role of mental health in physical wellbeing cannot be overstated. By nurturing our minds and bodies in harmony, we can unlock our full potential and achieve best health and fitness.

Let us embrace the power of positivity, mindfulness, and resilience in our workout journey, and strive towards a healthier and happier version of ourselves. Remember, you are capable of greatness, both mentally and physically.

Practicing Mindfulness and Stress Relief Techniques

Practicing mindfulness and stress relief techniques is essential for maintaining a healthy mind and body. In our fast-paced world, it can be easy to get caught up in the chaos and forget to take care of ourselves.

However, by incorporating simple mindfulness practices into your daily routine, you can reduce stress, improve mental clarity, and enhance your overall well-being. One effective way to practice mindfulness is through meditation.

Taking just a few minutes each day to sit quietly and focus on your breath can have a profound impact on your mental state. By centering yourself in the present moment, you can let go of worries about the past or future and experience a sense of calm and

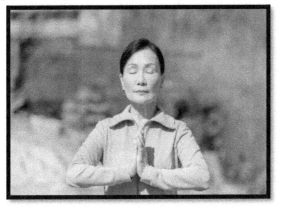

clarity.

Another powerful stress relief technique is exercise. Physical activity has been shown to reduce levels of the stress hormone cortisol and release endorphins, which are natural mood elevators. Our

Single Band Full-Body Workout is the ultimate way to get moving and release tension in your body.

By engaging in regular exercise, you can improve your physical health while also boosting your mental well-being. In addition to meditation and exercise, practicing gratitude can also help reduce stress and cultivate a positive mindset. Taking time each day to reflect on the things you are grateful for can shift your focus away from negativity and towards appreciation.

This Simple Practice Can Help You Feel More Content And At Peace With Your Life.

Remember, taking care of your mental health is just as important as taking care of your physical health. By incorporating mindfulness and stress relief techniques into your daily routine, you can improve your overall well-being and lead a happier, healthier life. Take some time each day to practice mindfulness, exercise regularly, and cultivate gratitude – your mind and body will thank you for it.

Incorporating Mindful Movement into Your Workouts

Incorporating mindful movement into your workouts can transform not only your physical fitness, but also your mental well-being.

By bringing awareness to each movement, you can deepen your connection to your body and deeply appreciate the power and strength it has. This subchapter will guide you on how to infuse mindfulness into your workouts, elevating your exercise experience to a whole new level. When you engage in mindful movement, you are fully present in the moment, focusing on the sensations in your body and the rhythm of your breath.

This awareness allows you to perform each exercise with intention and purpose, maximizing the benefits for your muscles and overall fitness. By being mindful, you can prevent injuries, improve your posture, and enhance your coordination and balance.

As you embark on your single band full-body workout, take a moment to set an intention for your session. Whether it's to build strength, increase flexibility, or simply enjoy moving your body, having a clear goal will keep you motivated and focused.

Throughout your workout, pay attention to how each movement feels in your body, adjusting as needed to ensure proper form and alignment. Mindful movement can also help you cultivate a sense of gratitude for your body and its capabilities. Instead of viewing exercise as a chore or a means to an end, see it as a gift that allows you to nourish and strengthen your body. By approaching your workouts with gratitude and appreciation, you can transform your relationship with exercise and create a positive and sustainable fitness routine. Incorporating mindful movement into your workouts is a powerful way to enhance your physical and mental well-being.

By bringing awareness to each movement, setting intentions, and cultivating gratitude, you can elevate your exercise experience and deepen your connection to your body. Embrace the power of mindfulness in your workouts and watch as it transforms not only your fitness journey, but also your overall outlook on health and wellness.

Chapter 7: Taking Your Fitness Journey to the Next Level

Exploring Different Types of Resistance Bands and Equipment

We investigate the world of resistance bands and equipment, exploring the several types available to enhance your workout routine. Resistance bands are versatile tools that can be used by teens, adults, and seniors to build strength, improve flexibility, and increase endurance. By incorporating these bands into your exercise regimen, you can take your fitness journey to the next level.

One of the most common types of resistance bands is the loop band, which provides continuous resistance throughout the movement. This band is ideal for targeting specific muscle groups and can be easily adjusted to increase or decrease the intensity of your workout. Another popular choice is the tube band, which comes with handles for a comfortable grip and allows for a wider range of motion.

Whether you are a beginner or a seasoned fitness enthusiast, there is a resistance band that suits your needs and preferences.

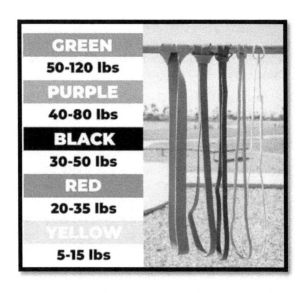

GREEN	50-120 lbs
PURPLE	40-80 lbs
BLACK	30-50 lbs
RED	20-35 lbs
YELLOW	5-15 lbs

In addition to resistance bands, there are various types of equipment that can be used to complement your workouts. From stability balls to kettlebells, each piece of equipment offers unique benefits for strengthening different muscle groups. By incorporating various equipment into your routine, you can challenge your body in new ways and prevent plateaus in your fitness progress.

As you explore the different types of resistance bands and equipment, remember that consistency is key to seeing results. Set realistic goals for yourself and stay committed to your workout plan. With dedication and perseverance, you can achieve your fitness goals and improve your overall health and

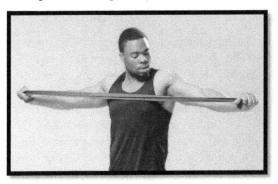

well-being. Embrace the challenge and push yourself to new heights with the help of these powerful tools.

Incorporating a variety of resistance bands and equipment into your workout routine can help you achieve a full-body workout that targets all major muscle groups. By exploring the diverse types of bands and equipment available, you can customize your workouts to suit your fitness level and goals.

Stay motivated, stay focused, and remember that every step you take towards a healthier lifestyle is a step in the right direction. Let the power of resistance bands and equipment propel you towards a stronger, fitter, and more confident version of yourself.

Research proper techniques and form on YouTube In this subchapter, we will delve into the world of YouTube to discover a wealth of information on proper techniques and form for your single band full-body workout. YouTube is a treasure trove of fitness resources, with countless videos proving exercises and providing valuable tips to ensure you are getting the most out of your workout routine.

By taking the time to research proper techniques and form on YouTube, you can enhance your workout experience and maximize your results. Whether you are a teen, adult, or senior, YouTube offers something for everyone when it comes to fitness. From beginner tutorials to advanced workout routines, there is no shortage of content to help you achieve your fitness goals. By immersing yourself in the world of fitness videos on YouTube, you will be inspired to push yourself further and challenge your body in new and exciting ways.

One of the key benefits of using YouTube to research proper techniques and form is the visual aspect. Watching demonstrations of exercises in real-time can be incredibly helpful in understanding how to perform them correctly.

This visual guidance can help prevent injury and ensure you are targeting the right muscle groups during your workout. By following along with knowledgeable fitness trainers on YouTube, you can learn the proper form for each exercise and make the most out of your single band full-body workout.

Furthermore, YouTube provides a platform for fitness enthusiasts to share their knowledge and ability with a global audience. By tapping into this vast network of trainers and experts, you can gain valuable insights and tips to improve your workout routine.

From tips on breathing techniques to advice on proper alignment, there is no shortage of information to help you perfect your form and technique. By staying informed and up to date on the latest fitness trends and techniques, you can stay motivated and inspired on your fitness journey.

In summary, using YouTube as a resource to research proper techniques and form for your single band full-body workout can be a meaningful change in your fitness journey. By immersing yourself in the world of fitness videos, you can gain valuable insights, tips, and inspiration to take your workout routine to the next level. Grab your band, fire up YouTube, and get ready to elevate your workout experience like never before. Remember, the key to success lies in proper technique and form – and YouTube is here to help you every step of the way.

Continuing to Grow and Evolve in Your Fitness Journey

As you embark on your fitness journey with the Single Band Full-Body Workout, it's important to remember that growth and evolution are key components of a successful fitness routine. Just as our bodies are constantly changing and adapting, so too should our workout plans. By continuing to challenge yourself and push beyond your comfort zone, you will not only see physical changes in your body, but you will also experience personal growth and development. One of the most important aspects of continuing to grow and evolve in your fitness journey is setting goals for yourself. Whether it's increasing the number of reps you can do with a certain exercise, improving your flexibility, or reaching a specific weight loss target, having clear and achievable goals will keep you motivated and focused.

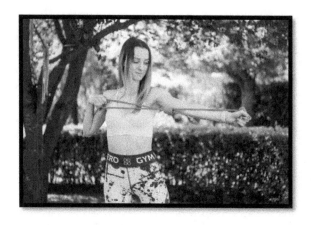

Remember, progress is not always linear, so don't get discouraged if you hit a plateau. Instead, use it as an opportunity to reassess your goals and push yourself even further. Another key to growth and evolution in your fitness journey is variety. While the Single Band Full-Body Workout provides a comprehensive and effective workout plan, it's critical to mix things up occasionally. Try incorporating new exercises, changing up your routine, or increasing the intensity of your workouts. This will not only prevent boredom, but it will also challenge different muscle groups and help you continue to see progress.

Consistency is also crucial when it comes to growing and evolving in your fitness journey. Make a commitment to yourself to stick to your workout plan and make healthy choices every day. Remember, results don't happen overnight, so be patient and stay dedicated to your goals. Celebrate your achievements, no matter how small, and use them as motivation to keep pushing forward.

Your fitness journey is a lifelong process of growth and evolution. By setting goals, incorporating variety, staying consistent, and pushing yourself beyond your limits, you will continue to see progress and achieve your fitness goals. Remember, it's not just about physical changes, but also about personal growth and development. Embrace the journey, stay positive, and keep challenging yourself to become the best version of yourself.

Embracing the Journey of One Band, One Body

Embracing the journey of one band, one body is not just about physical exercise, it is about empowering yourself to be the best version of yourself. Through this workout plan, you can strengthen not only your muscles but also your mind and spirit. It is an integrated approach to fitness that will help you achieve your goals and live a healthier, happier life. As you continue this journey, remember that consistency is key.

Results may not come overnight, but with dedication and perseverance, you will see progress. Trust the process and believe in yourself. You have the power to transform your body and your life through the power of one band and one body. One band, one body is not just a workout plan, it is a lifestyle. It is about making healthy choices every day and prioritizing your well-being.

By committing to this program, you are taking a step towards a stronger, fitter, and more confident you. Embrace the journey and enjoy the transformation that comes with it.

Remember, you are not alone on this journey. Surround yourself with a supportive community of like-minded individuals who are also striving for greatness. Share your successes and challenges and celebrate each other's victories.

Together, we can achieve remarkable things and inspire each other to reach new heights. In closing, I encourage you to continue embracing the journey of one band, one body with enthusiasm and determination. Be proud of how far you have come and excited for what lies ahead. With dedication, perseverance, and a positive attitude, you can achieve anything you set your mind to. Believe in yourself, trust the process, and let the power of one band and one body guide you towards a healthier, happier you. I have many more band and isometric exercises on my blog. isoquickstrength.blogspot.com

Printed in the USA
CPSIA information can be obtained
at www.ICGtesting.com
LVHW011916101124
796066LV00015B/796